PRACTICAL GUIDE TO YOGA

PRACTICAL GUIDE TO YOGA

[ILLUSTRATED]

Sri Swami Chidananda

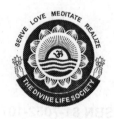

Published by

THE DIVINE LIFE SOCIETY
P.O. SHIVANANDANAGAR—249 192
Distt. Tehri-Garhwal, Uttarakhand, Himalayas, India

Price]   2008   **[Rs. 40/-**

First Edition: 1977
Eleventh Edition: 2008
[2,000 Copies]

©The Divine Life Trust Society

ISBN 81-7052-107-6
EC34

Published by Swami Vimalananda for
The Divine Life Society, Shivanandanagar, and
printed by him at the Yoga-Vedanta Forest Academy
Press, P.O. Shivanandanagar, Distt. Tehri-Garhwal,
Uttarakhand, Himalayas, India

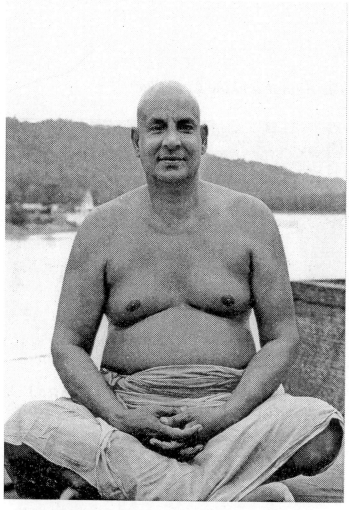

H.H. SRI SWAMI SIVANANDAJI MAHARAJ

(Founder—The Divine Life Society)

The Author and the Compiler:

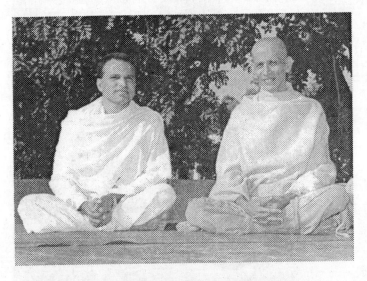

**SRI SWAMI CHIDANANDAJI MAHARAJ
WITH SRI SWAMI YOGASWARUPANANDA**

(Formerly known as Sri Krishnamurthy)

SRI SWAMI CHIDANANDA

AN APOSTLE OF PEACE AND EMBODIMENT OF QUINTESSENCE OF INDIA'S SPRITUAL AND CULTURAL HERITAGE

Revered Gurudev Swami Sivanandaji's worthy spiritual successor has been referred to as follows, "If one wants to see boldness of spirit behind a slender appearance, irrevertible command of heart behind a benign face, unwavering peace of mind behind dynamism of action, impersonal detachment behind personal love and care—all at once in a single person, one cannot do better than meet Swami Chidananda."

Born on 24th September, 1916, into a wealthy Brahmin family in South India, Swami Chidananda absorbed love for tradition and respect for rituals. At Loyola College, Madras (now Chennai), Swamiji had a brilliant scholastic career. The ideals and teachings of Jesus made a deep impression in his heart, and he was able to synthesize them with all that is best and noble in Hindu Culture. The two profound influences in Swamiji's life were the teachings of Sri Ramakrishna and the example of his Gurudev, Sri Swami Sivananda. He joined Gurudev in 1943 and from then on the Ashram and the lofty ideals of The Divine Life Society became home and field of service for him.

Swami Chidananda was born with an insatiable zeal to serve the sick and the suffering. Even in childhood he built huts for lepers on the lawns of his home and looked after them as though they were deities.

Swami Sivananda said about his spiritual son and beloved disciple:

"Chidananda is a Jivanmukta, a great Saint, an ideal Yogi, a Para-Bhakta and a great sage. Swami Chidananda is all this and much more. He was a great Yogi and Saint in his previous birth itself. His lectures are the outpouring of his saintly heart, the revelations of intuitive wisdom. And he is a practical Vedantin, his words have tremendous power. He is born to fulfil a great mission."

Sri Swami Chidanandaji Maharaj attained Mahasamadhi on 28th August, 2008.

PUBLISHERS' NOTE

This book on Yoga physical exercises is perhaps the second publication by The Divine Life Society after the first and earliest work on Hatha Yoga and Asanas by Gurudev Sri Swami Sivanandaji Maharaj. The present work is a compilation by Sri Swami Yogaswarupanandaji (formerly known as Brahmachari Sri Krishnamurthyji) of the Ashram, who is a senior Sadhaka and a Hatha Yoga Instructor himself, of the practical instructions given on Hatha Yoga and Asanas by Revered Sri Swami Chidanandaji Maharaj.

As a first step on the path of Yoga Sadhana (spiritual practice), the necessity for physical fitness hardly needs any explanation. Even for a householder engaged in his daily activities, the necessity to keep the system physically fit to attend to his daily duties is quite obvious. Seen in this light, the present work which contains exposition on a set of select important Asanas which can be conveniently practised daily, not only by the whole-time spiritual Sadhakas but also by ordinary householders, is thus a boon to the aspirants treading the path of spiritual Sadhana and to the general public. The book answers many questions that may arise in the minds of the earnest aspirants, clears many of their doubts and removes unnecessary and unfounded fears that may lurk in them concerning possible harmful effects of practising Yoga Asanas. Revered Swamji has taken the pains of illustrating the postures with his own photographs and has given practical guidance in the technique of meditation which is the desired goal to which perfection in postures (Asana-Jaya) leads the practising seeker.

The value and benefit that will accrue by a study of this book is indeed considerable and great. We therefore have no doubt that the present publication will have a warm reception and wide circulation.

Shivanandanagar,
14th January, 1977

—THE DIVINE LIFE SOCIETY

INTRODUCTION

Salutations to the primal Yogishwara Lord Siva and to the Great World Teacher Yogeshwara Lord Krishna. Reverential prostrations at the feet of my Yogi Guru Late Revered Swami Sivanandaji Maharaj of sacred memory. My loving good wishes to all Yoga students upon the path of self-development for their fullest success in their Yoga practice.

It gives me much happiness to write this brief Introduction to this present book which is an excellent, hand manual for ready reference to all sincere students of the Yoga science. This book is specially meant to serve as a day-to-day home guide for those who are practising a daily course of Yoga Asanas for their physical and mental health, strength and well-being. Yoga is a system of physical, vital and mental culture and spiritual unfoldment. Much valuable information and instruction is contained in the pages of this volume regarding all aspects of daily Yoga Sadhana. The inclusion of Suryanamaskara as well as meditation will confer great deal of additional benefit to the reader. Well-selected illustrations further enhance the utility of this Yogi's Companion.

Study this volume completely from start to finish, when you take up the practice. Take special note of Chapters 1, 2, 3 and 21. Approach your daily practice with right attitude and spiritual Bhava. Proceed gradually. Do not go to extremes in your Yoga practice. There should be no hastiness. Keep your attention steadily fixed upon whatever posture or process you are doing at the moment. Such steady attention increases the value of the practice. Maintain a pleasant frame of mind. Be poised and relaxed. The Yoga practice place must always be clean, neat and tidy. The clothes you use and the blanket, etc., that you spread during the practice should not be used for other purposes. Please remember that Yoga is a sacred science and its practice is primarily a spiritual process though based upon physical body, breath and mind-control. Then you will be fortunate enough to obtain the maximum benefit from this science which is meant to help all mankind to attain health, peace and joy.

Be regular. Try to be punctual. Do perfectly even if you do only a little every day. If you have no time according to your present daily programme then I suggest that you wake up one hour earlier in the morning. This will give you an hour's time which is absolutely your own and when you are free to use it for Yoga. Observe the important instructions given in Chapter 3. Maintain sincere interest and steady enthusiasm. When you do the postures do not try to immediately assume it in its acute and extreme form. Gradually proceed until you master it in due course of time. This will save your body from too much extreme strain and the physical pains resulting from such strain. You must be wise and use your common-sense all throughout.

One word is necessary in connection with Yoga practice. There is a tendency nowadays to frighten Yoga students by alarming statements that practice of Yoga exercises may result in incurable diseases or other harmful effects to body and mind. Students are discouraged from taking to the practice by the statement that practice should be undertaken only under an expert and adept as otherwise harm would result. I wish to clarify this matter here. While it is true that for the *whole-timed practice* of Hatha Yoga or Kundalini Yoga as the main Sadhana of a Sadhaka it is imperative to have an adept Guru, nevertheless no such strict regulation applies to the practice of a select few Asanas and Pranayama undertaken as a daily health culture course by the ordinary layman. A short daily course of half-an-hour or one hour's practice of a select few postural exercises can be undertaken by any person in normal health without fear or risk of any sort of untoward harmful effect. On the contrary the results will be entirely beneficial, helpful and healthful. There is no need for any unnecessary baseless alarm or hesitation in taking up such a limited practice as a daily routine provided the instructions given in this connection are kept in mind and observed.

Swami Yogaswarupanandaji is mainly responsible for this careful compilation of the entire text of the book. I congratulate this very earnest student who has shown great sincerity in his pursuit of knowledge. The book is the result of his attentive hearing of my explanations and instructions during talks he had with me on Sadhana in general and on Yoga Asanas, Pranayama, etc., in particular. After attentive listening, he took down notes diligently and later developed them into this manuscript. I am very happy that the fruit of his labours now comes to all Sadhakas and students of Yoga in the form of this present compact and attractive volume which will prove of definite use to every student of Yoga. I wish this volume widest possible circulation and pray to the Lord to confer health, strength and success to all those who take up to the practice of Yoga.

Swami Chidananda

ॐ

PRAYERS

The first prayer is to be chanted before the commencement and the second one at the conclusion of the practice of Asanas.

I

ॐ सह नाववतु। सह नौ भुनक्तु। सह वीर्यं करवावहै
तेजस्विनावधीतमस्तु। मा विद्विषावहै॥
ॐ शान्तिः शान्तिः शान्तिः ॥

*Om Saha Navavatu Saha Nau Bhunaktu,
Saha Viryam Karavavahai,
Tejasvi Navadhitamastu Ma Vidvishavahai,
Om Santih Santih Santih!*

MEANING: Om! May He protect us both (the Teacher and the Taught). May He cause us both to enjoy protection. May we both exert to find out the true meaning of the scriptures. May what we study become lustrous. May we never quarrel with each other. Om Peace, Peace, Peace!

II

ॐ पूर्णमदः पूर्णमिदं पूर्णात्पूर्णमुदच्यते।
पूर्णस्य पूर्णमादाय पूर्णमेवावशिष्यते॥
ॐ शान्तिः शान्तिः शान्तिः ॥

Om Purnamadah Purnamidam
Purnat Purnamudachyate
Purnasya Purnamadaya
Purnamevavasishyate
Om Santih Santih Santih!

MEANING: The invisible (Brahman) is the full; The visible (the world) too is full. From the full (Brahman) the full (the visible universe) has come. The full (Brahman) remains the same even after the full (the visible universe) has come out of the full (Brahman). Om Peace, Peace, Peace!

CONTENTS

	Publishers' Note 8
	Introduction 10
	Prayers 14
1.	Purpose of Yoga. 21
2.	Benefits of Yogic Exercises 25
3.	Important Instructions. 27
4.	Preliminary Standing Postures 30
(1)	Tadasana 30
(2)	Trikonasana 31
(3)	Suryanamaskara 33
5.	Savasana 49
6.	Sirshasana 52
7.	Sarvangasana 56
8.	Matsyasana 58
9.	Halasana 60
10.	Paschimottanasana 62
11.	Bhujangasana 63
12.	Makarasana 65
13.	Salabhasana 66

14.	Dhanurasana	67
15.	Chakrasana	69
16.	Ardha-Matsyendrasana	70
17.	Yoga Mudra	71
18.	Mayurasana	73
19.	Sitting Postures	75
	(1) Padmasana	75
	(2) Siddhasana	76
	(3) Svastikasana	77
	(4) Vajrasana	78
20.	Pranayama	80
	(1) Deep Breathing Exercise	81
	(2) Kapalabhati	82
	(3) Bhastrika	83
	(4) Sitali	84
	(5) Sitkari	85
	(6) Ujjayi	86
	(7) Sukha Purvaka	88
21.	Dhyana	91
22.	Conclusion	94
23.	Brief Life-Sketch of Sri Swami Chidananda	97

PRACTICAL GUIDE TO
YOGA

1. PURPOSE OF YOGA

Harmony is called Yoga—*Samatvam yoga uchyate,*—says the Bhagavadgita. In spite of all scientific advancement, even today man continues to suffer as before, from the beginning of recorded history. This is due to disharmony within himself and with the world outside. Man is nothing but a part of Nature. And Nature is constituted and governed by the three Gunas, the fundamental entities, Tamas, Rajas and Sattva. The 'Gunas' here do not mean properties or characteristics. They are the substances out of which this universe manifests itself in its multitudinous forms. Tamas is said to be static. Rajas, dynamic, and Sattva a state which is neither and which transcends the two. The process of evolution also is carried on by these three Gunas. Evolution means creation and its progressive development. Its basis lies in activity. These three Gunas exist like the three strands of a rope supporting one another. But, one Guna always predominates keeping the other two under subjugation. Our body is predominated by Tamoguna. It is gross, inert and visible. Prana is predominated by Rajoguna. It is dynamic and we feel its existence due to the movements in our body. Mind is predominated by Sattvaguna. Our entire personality is nothing but the combination of body, Prana and mind. This combination we call 'I'. All our troubles are due to a disharmony among these three, the body, Prana and mind. It is this state of disharmony that puts man under the clutches of the three Gunas. A state of harmony frees him from their grip. Yoga brings about this harmony. It prescribes Asana (posture), Pranayama (regulation of breath) and Dhyana (concentration and meditation). Asana is for bringing about harmony in the body, Pranayama in Prana and Dhyana in the mind. The nature of Tamoguna is to check or retard, but it should not be thought that when the movement is upwards through Rajoguna, Tamoguna is absent. Any process however small it may be, needs a force to develop, another force to move it, and a third to check or maintain it. The force that develops is Sattvaguna, that which causes movement is Rajoguna, and that which checks or maintains is Tamoguna. No one Guna exists in isolation without the influence of the other two. A lotus kept in a pot of water is disturbed when the pot is distrubed. The disturbance of the pot is transmitted to the water which in turn transmits it to the lotus. Similarly, any disturbance to the body is carried to the Prana, which again communicates it to the mind. To keep up the stability of our whole personality, Yoga prescribes Asana, Pranayama and meditation.

Sages emphatically declare that Yoga alone can destroy all pains. *Yogo bhavati duhkkaha*— Yoga is the destroyer of pain—says the Bhagavadgita. There are many definitions for Yoga. Merely memorising them and repeating them will not produce the desired result. Instead, we have to put it into practice in our daily life. If one understands the principles and applies them in one's day-to-day activities, life itself becomes a process of Yoga, and Yoga is the destroyer of pain.

Practice of Yoga creates harmony in the physical, vital, mental, psychological and spiritual aspects of the human personality. Different limbs constitute the human body. Similarly, there are a number of limbs in Yoga. They are mainly classified under eight heads:

Yama (moral restraints), *Niyama* (spiritual observances), *Asana* (posture), *Pranayama* (regulation of breath), *Pratyahara* (withdrawal of mind from external objects), *Dharana* (concentration on one object), *Dhyana* (meditation), and *Samadhi* (Supreme Harmony). If a person moves one step forward, all the limbs of the body also move simultaneously. Even so, if one practises even one limb of Yoga to a high degree of perfection, all the other limbs of Yoga are bound to accompany without great effort on the part of the practitioner.

When one desires to practise Yoga Asanas, one should naturally have externally congenial, conducive atmosphere. This can be brought about by observing *Yama*, viz., *Ahimsa* (observance of non-injury through thought, word and deed), *Satya* (truthfulness), *Brahmacharya* (all-round self-control), *Aparigraha* (non-acceptance of free gifts which are not essentials), *Asteya* (non-stealing). One should not practise Yoga Asanas when the mind is disturbed due to fear, anxiety, fatigue or tiresomeness. These can be overcome by the practice of Yama. An external congenial atmosphere alone is not sufficient. There must also be the internal serenity of mind. This is obtained by the practice of *Niyama*. This constitutes *Saucha* (internal and external purity), *Santosha* (contentment), *Tapas* (austerity), *Svadhyaya* (self-study) and *Isvarapranidhana* (surrender to God). Thus *Yama* and *Niyama* are two important unavoidable prerequisites for the practice of Yoga. The third and fourth limbs of Yoga are *Asana* and *Pranayama*. During the practice of Asanas there should not be any rapid movements of the limbs of the body or jerks of the body. By this, the breathing process is regulated automatically. While doing the Yoga Asanas, the mind should not think of the programmes and engagements of the day or any other external object. One must withdraw the mind from all such thoughts. This is called *Pratyahara,* the fifth limb. Here, a question may arise: On what should one direct the mind, when it is withdrawn from external thoughts, for its very nature is to go outward? Hence, it is suggested by the adepts that while doing Asanas, one should concentrate one's mind on the relevant parts of the body according to the nature of the Asana practised. Keeping the mind on a particular object for a short time is *Dharana* or concentration. Continuous concentratiion, on the object for a long time is called meditation. *"Pratyaya ekatanata dhyanam."* Thus when all the seven limbs of Yoga are brought in, the eighth limb, *Samadhi* or Supreme Harmony results as a natural sequence. The practice of Yoga Asanas thus leads to this Supreme Harmony.

Even though the ancient sages have named several postures with the appellations of reptiles, birds and animals with which they had some resemblance, only human beings can practise Yoga Asanas, combining with them the eight limbs of Yoga, but not the other beings. Merely bending the body cannot constitute Yoga Asanas. In Yoga, there should be a blending of all the eight limbs. Hence, Sage Patanjali said: *"Yoganga anushthanad asuddhi-kshaya jnana-diptir aa viveka khyateh*—By observing the eight limbs of Yoga, one effects the destruction of impurities, then arises spiritual illumination which leads into awareness of the Reality." This is the supreme purpose for which the practice of Yoga is recommended.

2. BENEFITS OF YOGIC EXERCISES

Good health is the greatest asset. Without good health one can hardly expect success in any walk of life. To keep up good health, there are numerous modern physical culture systems designed to develop the muscles. The physical culturist develops them by mechanical movements and exercises. In such physical exercises, there is a fast movement of the muscles resulting in the rapid functioning of the heart and lungs. The practitioner becomes exhausted very quickly. There may also be anxiety, psychological tension and fear. Some exercises develop the chest and the arms only, which becomes lopsided and results in disharmony in the personality.

In Yogic exercises, there is harmonious development of all the muscles of the body, internal organs, nerves and the frame. There are no rapid movements and hence there is no waste of energy. In Yoga exercise movements are gentle and rhythmic. On the other hand, they conserve energy.

The three important organs, viz., heart, lungs and brain with its cerebro-spinal system, are kept in a healthy condition by regular practice of a few important Asanas and one or two breathing exercises. Sound functioning of the organs depends upon good healthy nerves. The tripod of life are the brain, heart and the lungs. The heart and the lungs are under the control of the brain. These three important organs along with the cerebro-spinal system are kept in a healthy condition by regular Yogic exercises.

If the muscles are not given proper exercises, they will tend to contract and there will be stiffness and heaviness in the body. Blood circulation and nerve force will consequently be impeded. Their malfunctioning will disturb the organs. Some of the Yogic exercises concentrate on the development of the muscle also, consistent with the development of other parts as well.

These Yogic exercises are both preventive and curative in their nature. On the whole, they prevent diseases attacking the body by maintaining the natural health. Some exercises also cure existing diseases like cold, cough, constipation and gastric troubles.

Some Yogic exercises involve forward and backward motions, others help the lateral movement of the spine. Some clean the lungs, throat, etc. Thus the body as a whole is developed, toned up and strengthened. The entire body becomes flexible, thereby preventing stagnation of blood in any part of the body. Another unique feature of these exercises is, however, their influence upon the endocrine system of glands, the ductless glands as they are called. The malfunctioning of the thyroid, pituitary and pineal glands is corrected by a course of selected postures. Besides all this, some the exercises have great effect upon man's mind, his power of concentration and memory. They also wake up his dormant spiritual faculty. The Prana or the vital force is externalised in modern physical exercises, whereas the Yogic exercises make the Pranic current flow inwards. These Yogic exercises help to improve the health by regulating the functioning of the internal organs. Their regular practice brings to every practitioner, good health, longevity, strength, vim and vitality. By practising the Yoga Asanas regularly with care and caution, the personality as a whole will become pleasing and attractive.

This system is simple, exact, efficacious, economical and capable of being practised without any extraneous help when once a preliminary knowledge about it is obtained.

3. IMPORTANT INSTRUCTIONS

A word of warning and caution. There are certain 'dos' and 'dont's' here which should be adhered to at any cost, to derive maximum benefits and avoid harmful results by the practice of Yoga:

1. Generally, Yoga Asanas may be practised by young people only after twelve years of age, and not before. The minimum age limit is higher for certain specific Asanas like the Sirshasana and Sarvangasana. (see 'caution' under these Asanas).

2. Practice of Asanas for curing diseases must be done under the personal supervision of an experienced instructor.

3. Those who are suffering from chronic eye disease, running ears, high blood pressure and heart troubles should not practise Yoga Asanas. They can however practise relaxation in Savasana alone which is very beneficial to them.

4. Get up early in the morning at 4 or 4.30 a.m. If you feel sleepy, practise standing postures and four to six Suryanamaskaras. Then answer the calls of nature and wash your face.

5. If you are not in the habit of answering the calls of nature in the early morning, you can practise Asanas without answering the calls. After finishing the Asanas, Pranayama and meditation, you can go to the lavatory.

6. Take bath in luke warm water or cold water according to your capacity and convenience.

7. Wear a Langoti or Kowpina or suspendary bandage or close fitting underwear.

8. Spread a folded blanket on the floor and practise the Yoga Asanas over the blanket.

9. Do not wear spectacles or loose ornaments when you do Asanas. They may get damaged and may also cause injuries.

10. If you are accustomed to take bed-tea early in the mornings, after tea practise 4 to 6 Suryanamaskaras and then answer the calls of nature and start the practice.

11. Asanas should be done on empty stomach, in the morning, or at least 3 or 4 hours after food. Half an hour gap should be there before you take heavy tiffin or bath, after the practice of Asanas.

12. One cup of milk or tea can be taken ten minutes after the practice of Asanas. If before, then there must be an interval of at least half to one hour.

13. In the beginning, each Asana can be practised for a few seconds and gradually increase the duration of time. There should not be jerks or rapid movements of the body.

14. After the practice of Asanas and Pranayama, one must sit in a comfortable posture, and practise meditation at least for ten to thirty minutes, according to one's convenience.

15. If it is not possible to practise all the Asanas in the mornings, one can do the standing postures and Suryanamaskaras followed by Savasana. The remain-

IMPORTANT INSTRUCTIONS

ing Asanas and Pranayama can be practised in the evenings.

16. Before starting Sirshasana and also Pranayama, one must see that one's body and mind are calm, serene and undisturbed. If one is tired, fatigued, mentally or emotionally disturbed, then one should relax in Savasana for ten to fifteen minutes, and then start the practice.

17. Asanas should be practised in a well-ventilated clean room where there is free movement of fresh air. In cold regions, one can practise in a closed room. The floor must be even. Asanas can be practised on sandy river beds, open, airy places, and by the seaside.

18. If the practice of Asanas are discontinued due to some unavoidable circumstances there is no fear of any adverse reaction. After some days you can again start practising.

19. If you are a beginner, start the practice of Asanas from Sarvangasana onwards. Try Sirshasana after Yoga Mudra. Before Sirshasana, relax one or two minutes in Savasanas. While doing Sirshasana, the brain cells should be fresh without any fatigue or tiresomeness. The body must feel completely rested. Once you master the Sirshasana, then you can do it in the beginning itself, as per the sequence given in this book.

20. REGULARITY IS THE MOST IMPORTANT FACTOR IF YOU WANT TO DERIVE THE FULL BENEFITS OF THE YOGA ASANAS QUICKLY.

4. PRELIMINARY STANDING POSTURES

(1) TADASANA

(Mountain posture or standing posture)

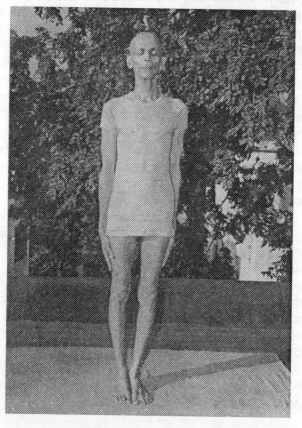

This is the basis for all standing postures. This may be taken as relaxation in a standing position.

TECHNIQUE

Stand in a straight posture by keeping the legs together, and also keep the big toes, heels and knees touching each other. Keep the hand fingers stretched by the side of the thigh muscles, and the chest forward. Entire weight of the body should rest evenly on the heels and toes. Breathing should be normal and slow. Close your eyes. Hear all the external sounds without resistance, and be one with nature.

BENEFITS

One will feel lightness in the body due to equal distribution of the weight on the heels and toes of the two legs. The mind acquires calmness due to uniform flow of Prana in the body.

(2) TRIKONASANA

(Triangle Posture)

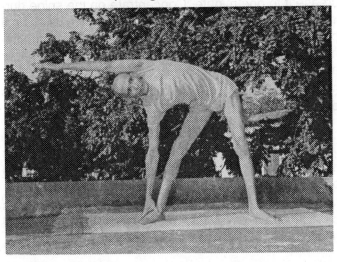

In the Trikonasana there is a lateral movement of the spine, whereas in Suryanamasakara there are forward and backward movements of the spine. Thus by practising these standing postures, the spine becomes more flexible. Flexibility is the symptom of young age.

TECHNIQUE

Stand in Tadasana. Separate your legs and keep them 2 to 2½ feet apart. Slowly stretch both the hands to the level of the shoulders with palms facing down and keep them parallel to the ground. Slowly exhale and bend the trunk towards the right and try to keep the right palm touch the ground near the right ankle, all the while keeping the legs straight without bend. The entire palm may be made to rest on the foot. Keep the left hand stretched over the head and parallel to the ground. Look forward. Retain the posture for a few seconds in the beginning, with normal breathing, and gradually increase it to one minute. Concentrate on the spine during this posture. Slowly bring the left hand to its original position, lift the right hand from the ground and simultaneously straighten the trunk and bring the legs together and stand erect in Tadasana.

After 2 or 3 deep breaths, repeat the process bending the trunk on the left side.

BENEFITS

This Asana removes the stiffness in the legs, arms and hips, corrects minor deformities in the legs, relieves backache and neck sprains, and develops the chest.

Note: Standing postures and Suryanamaskaras can be practised by all, young and old, with normal health, *without any age restrictions.*

(3) SURYANAMASKARA

The Suryanamaskara or offering prostrations to the Sun, is practised in the early morning or evening, facing the Sun. The Sun is supposed to be the deity for health and long life. The genius of the Indian sage has, in the Suryanamaskara Exercise, evolved a unique method of effecting perfect synthesis of culture of body, mind and spirit. With his intuitive insight into the nature of the mass mind, the Indian Sage has cleverly woven into every man's daily routine this unparalleled system of all-round self-culture.

A harmonious development of the body and mind alone can enable man to fulfil his ambitions and live a fruitful and happy life here in this world. A sickly body acts as a dead-weight preventing the mind from soaring into the higher realms. An excellent, well-built body, strong and healthy, if it serves only to house an undeveloped or diseased mind, is capable of much harm and little good to anyone. A good body, and a keen mind, with the inner spirit entirely dormant is like a lovely mansion without foundation liable to topple over at any moment. A perfectly harmonious development of the body, mind and spirit makes one perfect. Suryanamaskara achieves this harmonious development.

Suryanamaskara is combined process of Yoga Asanas and Pranayama (Yogic postures and regulated breathing). Before students take up the practice of more complicated and difficult Yogic postures and exercises in Pranayama, the spine and body muscles should acquire some flexibility. This exercise of

Suryanamaskara reduces abdominal fat, brings flexibility to the spine and limbs, and also increases the breathing capacity.

There are twelve spinal positions each stretching various ligaments and giving different movements to the vertebral column. The vertebral column is bent forward and backward alternately with deep inhalation and exhalation of breath and a little of retention of breath in some cases. Whenever the body is bent forward, the contraction of the abdomen and diaphragm, throws out the breath. When the body bends backward the chest expands and deep inhalation occurs automatically. In this way the body becomes flexible and the entire portion of the lungs begins to function which results in correct breathing. Moreover, it gives mild exercises to leg and arm muscles and ensures good circulation of blood. At the same time, the sun's life-giving rays play on the man's body, sucking away the toxins along with perspiration invigorating circulation and imparting life to the human organism—the life which the sun alone can give. For a person with stiff limbs and spine the Suryanamaskara exercise is a boon to bring back lost flexibility.

TECHNIQUE

Caution: During all these positions, movements of the limbs and breathing must be very, very slow and rhythmical. Sudden jerks of any part of the body and hard inhalation and exhalation in quick succession including retention of breath causing strain in the lungs, should be completely avoided.

PRELIMINARY STANDING POSTURES

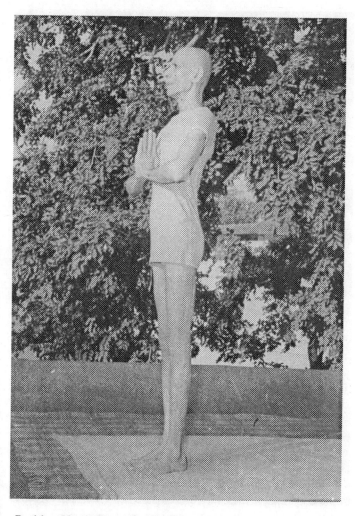

Position No. 1: Face the sun, fold the hands, keep the palms together touching the middle of the chest with both thumbs, keep legs together and stand erect.

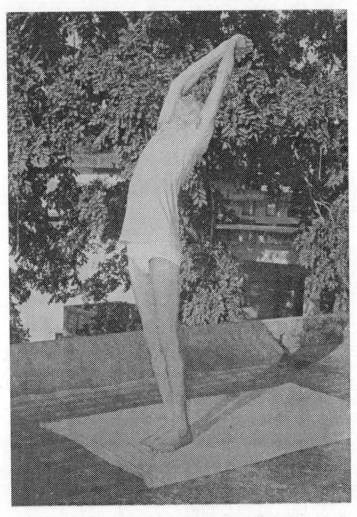

Position No. 2: **Slowly inhale and raise the arms overhead. Bend backward.**

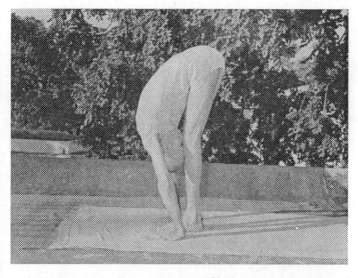

Position No. 3: Slowly exhale and bend forward till the palms are kept flat in line with the feet. Touch the knees with your head keeping the legs straight without bending. In the beginning there may be slight bend at the knees to effect this, but after some days' practice, the legs could be kept straight.

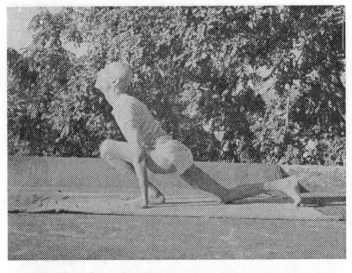

Position No. 4: After slow and deep inhalation, move the right leg from the body in a long backward step. Keep the hands and the left foot firmly on the ground without moving, raise the head, and look forward. The left knee should be between the hands.

PRELIMINARY STANDING POSTURES 39

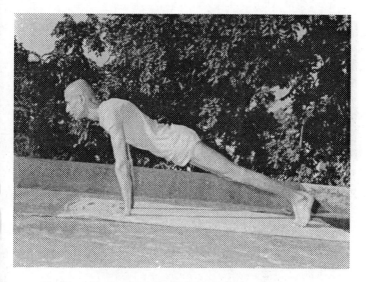

Position No. 5: Retain the breath. Move the left leg
and keep the left foot along with the right foot,
thus making the body a straight line.
The entire weight of the body should rest
on the hands and toes.

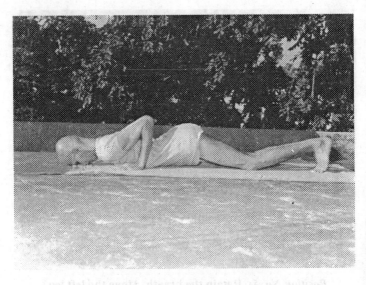

Position No. 6: **Exhale, slowly lower the body and let eight limbs of the body—two toes, two knees, two hands, chest and forehead—alone touch the floor. The abdominal region is to be kept slightly raised.**

PRELIMINARY STANDING POSTURES 41

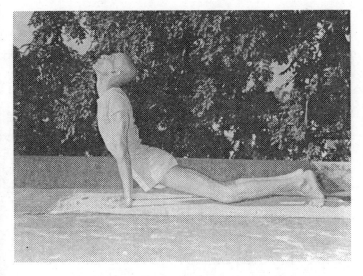

Position No. 7: With inhalation, slowly raise your head and bend the spine backward as much as possible.

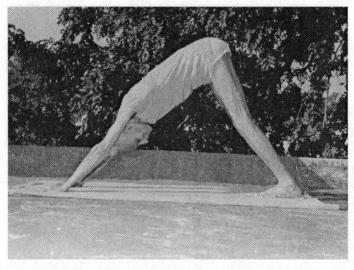

Position No. 8: **Exhale, slowly lower your head and raise the body, the toes and hands resting on the floor.**

PRELIMINARY STANDING POSTURES 43

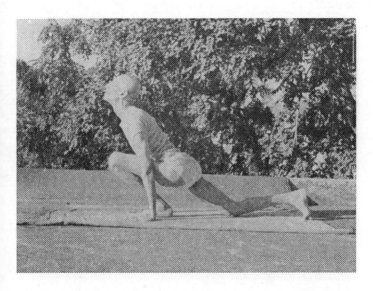

Position No. 9: Inhale and bring the left foot along the level of the hands. The right foot and knee should touch the ground. Look forward (Same as Position No. 4).

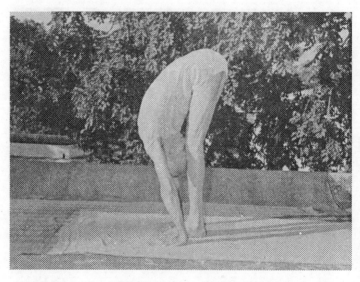

Position No. 10: **Exhale, bring the right leg also forward and come back to Position No. 3.**

PRELIMINARY STANDING POSTURES 45

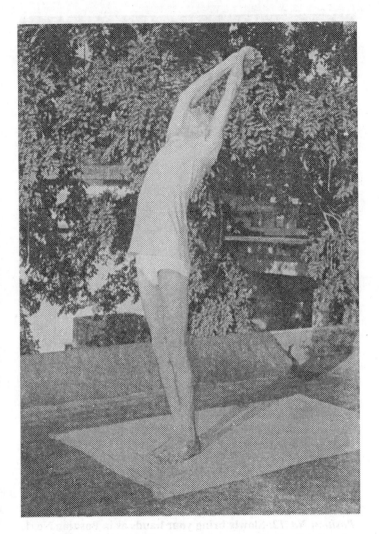

Position No. 11: Inhale and raise the hands overhead and bend backward as in Position No. 2.

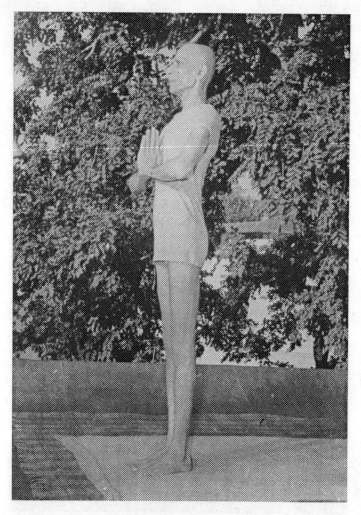

Position No. 12: Slowly bring your hands as in Position No. 1. Simultaneously exhale and relax in Tadasana.
This is one Namaskara.

PRELIMINARY STANDING POSTURES

After completing twelve *namaskaras* lie down flat on the ground on your back and relax each and every limb one by one from toes to the crown of the head. This is called Savasana (corpse pose). To begin with if one feels tired after three or four Namaskaras, he may stop with that and increase the number gradually (one everyday or every two days) all the time taking care that too much strain is not caused on any account, on any part of the body. The number may be increased according to each one's capacity. There are persons who can do 108 Namaskaras at a stretch without great strain.

Those who are spiritually or religiously inclined, would do well to follow, in addition, the instructions given below:

Before doing the Suryanamaskara the student may chant the prayer to the Almighty Lord:

PRAYER TO THE SUN

"Om Suryam Sundaralokanathamamritam
Vedantasaram Sivam,
Jnanam Brahmamayam Suresamamalam
Lokaikachittam Svayam;
Indradityanaradhipam Suragurum
Trailokyachudamanim,
Brahmavishnusivasvarupahridayam
Vande Sada Bhaskaram."

Meaning: I always adore Surya, the sun, the beautiful Lord of the world, the immortal, the quintessence of the Vedanta, the auspicious, the absolute knowledge, of the form of Brahman, the Lord of the gods, ever-pure, the one true consciousness of the world itself, the Lord of Indra, the gods and men, the preceptor of the gods, the crest-jewel of the three worlds, the very heart of the forms of Brahma, Vishnu and Siva, the giver of light.

Then repeat the twelve Names of the Lord by turn (mentally) for each Namaskara. The twelve names are:

1. *Om Mitraya Namah* (Prostration to Him who is affectionate to all).

2. *Om Ravaye Namah* (Prostration to Him who is the cause for change).

3. *Om Suryaya Namah* (Prostration to Him who induces activity).

4. *Om Bhanave Namah* (Prostration to Him who diffuses Light).

5. *Om Khagaya Namah* (Prostration to Him who moves in the sky).

6. *Om Pushne Namah* (Prostration to Him who nourishes all).

7. *Om Hiranyagarbhaya Namah* (Prostration to Him who contains everything).

8. *Om Marichaye Namah* (Prostration to Him who possesses rays).

9. *Om Adityaya Namah* (Prostration to Him who is the son of Aditi).

10. *Om Savitre Namah* (Prostration to Him who produces everything).

11. *Om Arkaya Namah* (Prostration to Him who is fit to be worshipped).

12. *Om Bhaskaraya Namah* (Prostration to Him who is the cause of lustre).

The sun being the most effulgent and life-giving force in this planet, it forms visible representation of the invisible Almighty Lord. The vast majority of men cannot think of the transcendent Supreme Absolute without the help of some concrete object or idea. To them the Sun forms the best object for worship and meditation.

Thus, Suryanamaskara provides the foundation for the magnificent all-round culture of body, mind and Spirit, which is essential for every human being.

5. SAVASANA OR MRITASANA

(Relaxation posture)

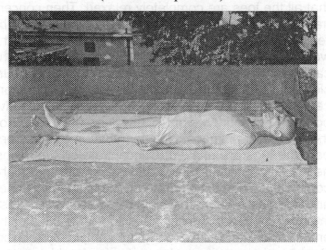

Now, you are going to relax wholly. Whatever strain, tension, or exertion is in the body, that is to be eliminated completely in this posture which is called Savasana.

Savasana combines pose with meditation. It gives rest not only for the body, but also for the mind. It gives relief, comfort and ease. Relaxation is a very important factor in muscular exercises.

TECHNIQUE

Lie down on your back, keep your hands by the side of your thighs with the palms facing upwards. Keep the legs apart without touching one another. Close your eyes.

Concentrate on the toes of both the feet, slightly move them and then relax. Now, mentally disconnect yourself from that part of the body, i.e., give the auto-suggestion: 'Let the toes go from my mind'. Feel that all the toes are completely relaxed. Then concentrate on the heels. The heavy weight of the legs will be resting on them. Relax the heels and relieve them of the weight, and feel they are relaxed. Concentrate on the calf muscles, relax them. Feel that up to the calf muscles both the legs are completely relaxed. Then concentrate on the knees which are nothing but heavy bones. The entire weight of the legs are resting on them. Relax the knees. Now feel that up to the knees both the legs are relaxed. Concentrate on the thighs, heavy muscles and bones and relax both the thighs completely. Then concentrate on the hip, heavy bones and muscles. The entire weight of the body will be resting on them. Relax the hips. Feel that up to the hip, the entire lower parts of the body are completely relaxed. Once you relax a particular part, you should not have any control over that part of the body. Now, concentrate on the vertebral column. The entire weight of the body will be resting on it. Relax the vertebral bones, one by one. Slowly relax up to the neck. Concentrate on the stomach and relax the stomach muscles completely. Feel the slight movement of the abdomen due to slow breathing. Concentrate on the chest. Feel that the entire weight of the chest is resting on the ribs. Relax the ribs and the chest. Breathe slowly and feel the harmonious movement of the lungs. Due to complete relaxation, feel that the entire chest region is becoming very light. Concentrate on the shoulders. The heavy weight of the body will be resting on the back of the shoulders. Relax the shoulders, biceps, elbows, forearms, wrists, palms and fingers. Feel that both the hands are completely relaxed. Now, concentrate on the neck. The heavy weight of the head is resting on the neck. Relax your neck. Slowly turn your head towards the right side. Slowly move it and bring it back to the centre. Turn your head towards the left side and slowly roll it and bring it back to the centre. Relax your neck completely. Concentrate on your head. Relax the head. Concentrate on your face and relax the face muscles. Concentrate on the lips, separate the lips slightly and relax them. Separate the two rows of the teeth and relax them. Just loosen your tongue and then relax it. Gently smile and relax the cheeks. Concentrate on the nostrils, breathe slowly and feel the slight movement of air through the nostrils. Relax the nostrils. Concentrate on the region of the eyes. Slowly and gently open the eyes partially, look at the sky (or roof), and then slowly close your eyes. The eye balls behind the eyelids may be gently directed downwards within. Relax the eyeballs. Let the eyes rest in perfect repose. Relax the eyebrows. Feel that the entire region of the eyes is completely relaxed. Concentrate on the forehead. Forget all other engagements. Have no thoughts in the mind. Feel that the entire forehead is relaxed. Concentrate on the ears. Hear the sound that come without resistance. Do not think of the nature, cause, etc., of the sounds. Be a witness to the sounds. Concentrate on the crown of your head. Feel a slight warmth there at the crown. Relax the head totally.

Feel that the heavy weight of the body is resting on the planet earth. Relax your body totally. Breathe gently in and out. Let the diaphragm be relaxed. Feel that the body is becoming lighter and lighter and it is floating in the space, in the ether. Feel also that is nothing but a centre of consciousness moving in space. This is our essential nature. Relax in this pose for a few minutes.

Now, slowly inhale and feel that fresh oxygen is entering and rejuvenating all the parts of the body. Exhale and feel that all the impurities are going out of the body. Once again, inhale and feel that fresh oxygen is entering and rejuvenating all the blood cells of the body; and then exhale and feel that all the impurities are going out.

With a deep inhalation, raise both the hands and place them on the ground above the head. Stretch your body from the toes to the tip of the hands. Turn your entire body from the toes up to the hands towards right, stretch the body and look at the hands. Bring the body back to the original position. Repeat the same process towards the left side. Slowly bring the hands by the side of the thighs. Slowly get up and sit, for a few seconds. Then, stand up on your toes and fully stretch the hands over the head. Slowly bring the hands down and relax. This whole process constitutes Savasana or complete relaxation.

6. SIRSHASANA

(Topsy-turvy posture)

TECHNIQUE

Sit on your knees before a fourfold blanket spread on the floor. Interlock your fingers making the palms of

SIRSHASANA

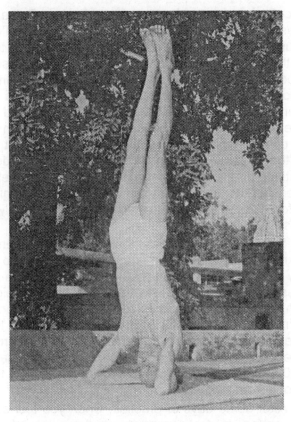

your hand to assume the form of a cup. Adjust the little fingers so that both palms may rest evenly on the blanket. Place the hands on the blanket, the little fingers touching the blanket. The line joining the elbows would be the base of the triangle now formed by the position of the hands on the blanket. The space between the elbows should be within the width of your chest. Next, place the crown of your head on the blanket so that the back of the crown touches the cupped palms. Raise the knees from the ground and keep the toes on the floor. Secure the position of your head, and bring the toes and thighs nearer to the body. Draw the knees close to the body and slowly raise the toes of the two legs simultaneously just off the floor and try to balance for a few seconds. When the balance becomes steady and the spine erect, straighten the knees and stretch both the legs up slowly bringing the whole body to a straight line with the head down and the feet high up. Do slow, deep breathing through the nose while in this posture. Retain the posture as long as you can without any discomfort, say for 10 to 15 seconds to start with, and gradually increase the period to 3 minutes.

Slowly exhale and lower the legs, bending them at the knees. Slowly draw the knees forward, close to the body and let the toes touch the floor. Straighten the knees with the toes on the floor and spine straight. Then, rest the knees on the floor and release the pose, placing the forehead so as to rest on your closed fists placed one upon the other. Remain in this position for 30 seconds and then stand on your legs (in Tadasana) for 30 seconds. This will prevent a sudden reverse flow of blood from the head.

After some days of practice, when you feel ease and comfort, try to concentrate on the crown of your head with normal breathing.

This Asana can be practised according to one's capacity and the duration may vary from one minute to three minutes for daily practice.

Note: Beginners should not stand on this pose too long. Avoid straining the body. When you feel any discomfort return to the normal position and relax. During the practice, mentally visualise the body, keeping the knees and toes straight but relaxed. Adjust your hands in such a way that the entire weight of the body should rest only on the head, but not on the hands. In the beginning, the sudden heavy flow of fresh blood into the head may cause some unusual feelings which you would gradually overcome and you would then feel comfortable. As you gain mastery, you would feel the body very light and at ease.

BENEFITS

Steady practice of Sirshasana makes the neck, stomach walls and thighs strong and powerful. The vertebral column is toned up and rendered strong. Regular practice of this Asana ensures proper flow of healthy and pure blood through all the body cells, especially in those parts above the heart, thus rejuvenating those parts. The thought-power also increases and thereby thoughts become more clear. The pituitary and pineal glands in the brain get proper blood supply and this ensures promotion of good health, growth and vitality. This Asana is specially beneficial to people suffering from loss of sleep, memory and vitality. Proper and correct practice of this Asana provides abundant energy and alertness. The lungs build up power to resist variations in climatic conditions, and makes one free from colds, coughs, tonsillitis, foul breath, palpitations, etc. It regulates the body temperature, removes constipation and tones up the blood content. Regular and correct practice also ensures proper and sound development of the body and mind. The power of concentration is increased.

Caution: High and low blood pressure patients and those suffering from heart troubles, pus in the ears, displaced retina and other chronic eye diseases, should not do this Asana. Children below *15 years* of age also must refrain from practising this Asana.

7. SARVANGASANA

(All-members' posture or Shoulder stand)

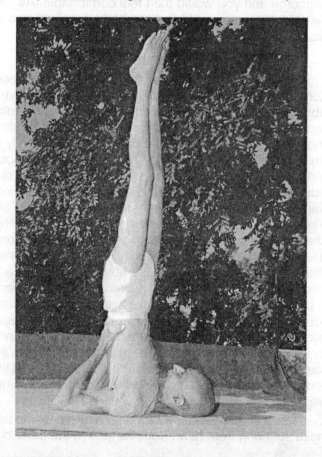

SARVANGASANA

TECHNIQUE

Spread a thick blanket on the floor. Lie flat on your back with legs stretched out, heels and knees together and the hands close to the sides of the body, palms facing the floor. Slowly inhale and simultaneously raise the legs without bending the knees. Slowly lift the trunk and support it at the back (in the middle of the spine) with your hands, bent at the elbows. Keep the spine vertical i.e., perpendicular to the floor. The back of the shoulders, neck and the back of the crown of the head should touch the floor, and the chin kept pressed tightly against the chest. When you get the spine vertical and establish balance in the posture, slowly stretch the legs with the toes pointing up. Keep the legs, the back and the spine in a straight line, vertical, in a relaxed position, with normal breathing.

Concentrate on the throat where fresh blood is flowing abundantly which promotes the secretion of the thyroid and para-thyroid glands. This is most important.

Exhale slowly, lower the legs without jerks and release the position of the hands. One should not lift the head from the ground while lowering the legs to its original position. Slowly slide down and lie flat and relax in Savasana for a few minutes. The duration for this posture may vary from one minute to three minutes for daily practice

BENEFITS

During the practice of this Asana, every part of the body is given exercise. Circulation of blood is directed to the thyroid and para-thyroid glands of the endocrine system. It stretches and renders pliable the muscles of the shoulders and the ligaments of the cervical region.

It helps the victims of varicose veins. It strengthens the muscles of the back and neck. It tones up arm muscles, and the body on the whole. It also checks elimination of toxin forming waste matter and regulates the entire blood circulation of the body.

Caution: As in Sirshasana.

8. MATSYASANA

(Fish posture)

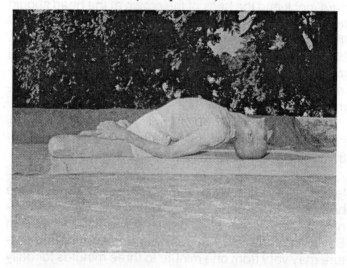

This Asana should be done immediately after Sarvangasana. The duration prescribed is one-third of the time for Sarvangasana. If one does the Sarvangasana for three minutes, this should be done for one minute. In this posture, one will derive some of the benefits of Sirshasana and Sarvangasana. In Sarvangasana there is a forward bend of the throat region, while here in this pose the neck region is stretched backward, so that fresh blood from the heart can flow abundantly to the brain where the pituitary and pineal glands are situated. During the practice of this Asana, the apices of the lungs (upper portion of the lungs) begin to function without any exertion to the body. Generally, this can be effected only after considerable physical exertion.

TECHNIQUE

Sit in Padmasana on a blanket spread on the floor. Slowly go back by resting on the elbows. Arch the back by lifting the chest and trunk and bend the neck backwards. Draw the head back and rest it on its crown. Raise your hands and catch hold of the big toes and gradually increase the arch by pressing further back the position of the crown of the head and pulling the toes by the hands. Concentrate on the chest, throat, crown of the head and the rear end of the spine, with normal breathing. Retain the posture for 20 seconds to one minute i.e., one-third duration of Sarvangasana. Release the toes by resting on the elbows and rest the back of your head on the ground. Slowly get up and sit in Padmasana and release the legs one by one.

As you gain mastery over this Asana, you may gradually increase the duration of the posture. Do slow, deep breathing while in posture.

Note: Beginners who are not in a position to sit in Padmasana, can stretch their legs and practise this Asana. The palms may rest on the thighs throughout.

BENEFITS

The chest and the dorsal regions are well expanded and breathing becomes more full. The pelvic joints are rendered more flexible. Due to the stretching of the neck, the thyroids are benefited. The spasm from the bronchial tubes are removed. This will effect some relief for the Asthma patients.

9. HALASANA

(Plough posture)

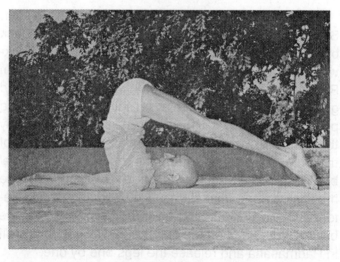

TECHNIQUE

Lie flat on your back with the arms at your sides and the palms resting on the ground. Keep your legs together, so that the big toe and the heel of one leg touch those of the other. Raise the legs slowly till they make a right angle with the trunk without bending the legs at the

HALASANA

knees. Keeping the hands on the ground, raise the hip and the lumbar part of the back also and bring down the legs to the floor beyond the head. Press the chin against the chest and breathe slowly through the nose. Let your palms, wrists and hands be kept flat on the floor. Lift your knees and stretch the toes as much as possible. Remain in this posture for a few seconds in the beginning with slow, deep breathing. Then, slowly raise the legs and bring them gradually, by degrees to the original posture of lying flat on the back. Gradually, increase the duration from one to three minutes, according to your capacity and convenience.

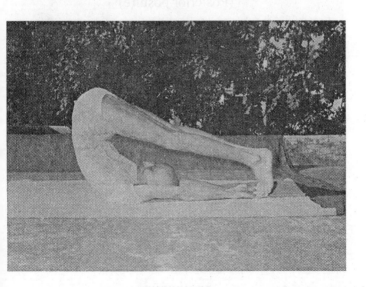

Variation: After lifting your knees and stretching the toes as much as possible, you may take the hands and catch hold of the toes.

BENEFITS

Various diseases and complications of the back, spine and shoulders and pains in the stomach and elbows are removed. The spine is rendered flexible and sturdy. The abdominal muscles get rejunvenated. Better blood circulation is effected into those parts of the abdominal organs, the spinal column, the back and the neck. This Asana reduces excess of fat from the abdomen, thighs and hips.

10. PASCHIMOTTANASANA

(Posterior posture)

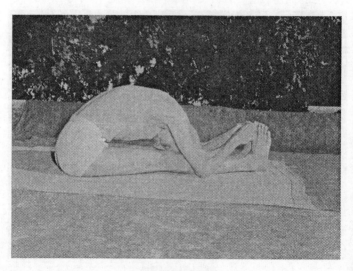

TECHNIQUE

Sit on a folded blanket with both the legs stretched and place the two hands on the knees. Slowly exhale, bend forward and catch hold of the big toes without lifting the knees. Bend your head down to touch the knees. Rest the elbows on the ground. Retain the posture for a few seconds. Gradually increase the duration of the time. Release the toes, and slowly return to the sitting position with inhalation. Take in a few slow deep breaths and exhale slowly. Repeat the posture two to three times. You can also do slow deep breathing while remaining in the posture.

When you gain mastery, you can comfortably stay for three to five minutes in the posture with normal breathing. While remaining in the posture, concentration should be on the spine and back muscles.

BENEFITS

Stiff back and all sorts of cramp in the back muscles, and other diseases of the back are cured. The elasticity of the spine is increased. The hamstring muscles behind the knees are strengthened. It removes sluggishness and tones up the kidneys and abdominal organs. It also rejuvenates the spine and promotes better digestion.

Note: In the case of many, perfection in this Asana can be achieved only by regular practice for a number of days. Care should be taken not to cause too much of strain to the hip region.

11. BHUJANGASANA

(Serpent posture)

TECHNIQUE

Lie prone on the ground with your forehead touching the ground. Place the palms down, on the floor below the shoulders. Keep the elbows close to the body.

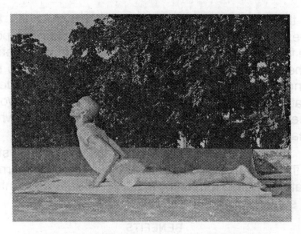

Keep the knees together. Extend the toes back, pointing them to the rear. Pressing the palms hard against the floor, inhale and slowly raise the upper part of the body. Draw the head far back feeling the vertebrae bend one by one, until the body from the navel downwards alone touches the floor. Feel that the entire weight of the body is resting on the legs and hip (rear end of the spine). No weight of the body should be on the palms. Retain the pose as long as possible (from 20 to 30 seconds). Concentrate on the abdomen and the rear end of the spine. Slowly lower the body and exhale. Release the entire body to rest on the floor and relax with deep breathing. Repeat the posture three times.

Finally, relax in *Makarasana* (*see* next posture).

BENEFITS

This Asana tones up the spine and expands the chest. It also helps to set right minor spinal disorders. The abdominal and back muscles get themselves well stretched, thereby effecting proper circulation of blood into the regions of the spinal column, stomach and back. It helps to increase the body-heat, promotes good appetite, removes constipation and increases the digestive power. This Asana specially renders the spine supple and elastic. This means providing of good health, vitality and juvenility to the individual.

This Asana is particularly helpful for ladies in toning up the ovaries and uterus.

12. MAKARASNA

(Crocodile posture)

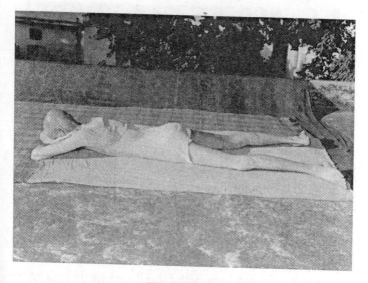

TECHNIQUE

Lie down face prone on the floor. Keep your crossed folded hands below the head, palms resting on the shoulders. Stretch the legs as far as possible, toes pointing outwards. Relax in this posture for two to three minutes, with normal breathing.

BENEFITS

The muscles that are put under severe strain demand relaxation and rest, and it is Makarasana that promptly and efficiently ensures complete relaxation and perfect ease to these muscles.

13. SALABHASANA

(Locust posture)

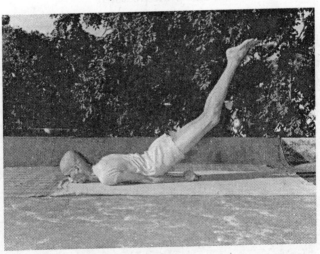

TECHNIQUE

Lie flat on the floor with face downwards and keep the hands by the side of the body with the fingers clenched into fists. Rest the chin on the ground by raising the head. Inhale and stiffen the body by pressing the fists against the floor. Slowly raise the legs as high as possible. Keep the legs in a straight line, while the two thighs, knees and ankles touch each other. The weight of the legs must fall on the body and hands. Contract the muscles of the buttocks, stretch the muscles of the thighs and further extend the position of the legs. Retain the posture for a few seconds in the beginning and gradually increase the duration. Concentrate on the upper portion of the body, i.e., above the waist. Slowly lower the legs to the floor and simultaneously exhale. Relax with normal breathing. Repeat the posture two or three times. Relax in Makarsana.

BENEFITS

The practice of this Asana renders the spine supple and elastic. It relieves backache or strain on the spine caused by hard work, etc. It also tones up the muscles at the back and the intestinal organs in the abdominal region and relieves pain in the lumbar and sacral regions. Above all it aids digestion and relieves gastric troubles.

14. DHANURASANA

(Bow posture)

TECHNIQUE

Lie flat, face downwards on the floor. Keep the hands at your side. Breathe out and bend the legs at the knees, drawing the feet above the thighs. Stretch the arms back and catch hold of the right ankle with the right hand and the left ankle with the left hand. Make secure the position of the hands, with normal breathing. Raise the head, body and knees by tugging the hands and legs, so that the whole weight of the body rests on

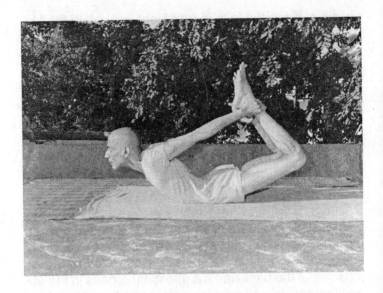

the abdomen. Retain the posture for a few seconds. Gradually increase the duration. While remaining in the posture, concentrate on the abdomen, thighs and back muscles. Release the ankles, stretch out the legs and bring the legs, chest and head to rest in a straight line on the floor. Relax in Makarasna for a few seconds. Repeat this Asana two or three times.

BENEFITS

This Asana relieves constipation and tones up the liver, pancreas and kidneys. The vertebrae of the lumbar and sacrum bones also get toned up. Proper blood circulation is effected and thus good health is promoted. This also renders the spine supple and elastic and minor pains in the spine are checked.

15. CHAKRASANA

(Wheel posture)

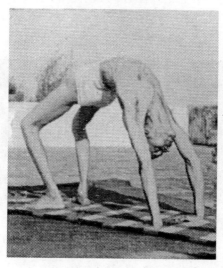

TECHNIQUE

Lie down on your back. Bend the legs at the knees and place the soles on the ground near the buttocks. Place the palms by the side of your head, fingers pointing towards the body. Slowly raise the body up by resting on the hands and feet, thus making a curve of your spine. Retain the posture for five seconds, and gradually increase the duration to one or two minutes. Concentrate on spine with normal breathing.

BENEFITS

All the benefits of Salabha, Bhujanga and Dhanurasanas are derived from this Asana. All parts of the body are given proper exercise during this posture.

16. ARDHA-MATSYENDRASANA

(Lateral spinal twist posture)

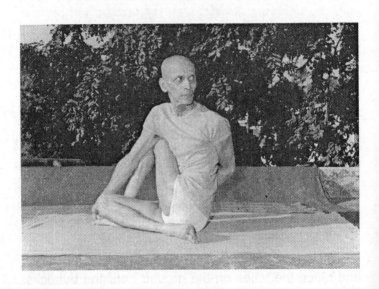

Matsyendra here refers to the Rishi or the teacher who first taught this Asana.

TECHNIQUE

Sit on the floor with legs stretched out. Bend the right leg at the knee and set the heel firmly against the perineum. Bend the left leg at the knee and lifting it from the floor with the support of the hands, place it by the side of the right thigh so that the left outer ankle touches the outer right thigh. Be secure in this position and keep the shin perpendicular to the floor. Now turn the trunk 90 degrees to the left, so that the right armpit touches the outer side of the left knee. Passing the right hand over the left knee, firmly catch hold of the left big toe with the right hand. Swing the left hand back and bring it round the right side of the waist to catch the right thigh. Turn the head over the left shoulder and direct the gaze over it. Give a full twist to the spine and stiffen the position. Retain the posture with normal breathing. Concentrate on the spine and the flow of breath. Remain in the posture for thirty seconds to one minute, and gradually increase to two to three minutes and then release. Repeat the same process by bending the left leg.

BENEFITS

A steady practice of this Asana cures lumbago and other muscular pains of the back. The spine is made elastic. The muscles and organs of the abdominal region are massaged. The roots of the nerves at the spine and the sympathetic system are toned up with a good supply of fresh and pure blood. Constipation and dyspepsia are removed. The nervous system and the vertebrae of the spinal column are given good exercise and they are toned up.

17. YOGA MUDRA

(Yogin's sealing posture)

TECHNIQUE

Sit on a folded blanket. Form a foot-lock by placing the right foot over the left thigh and left foot over the

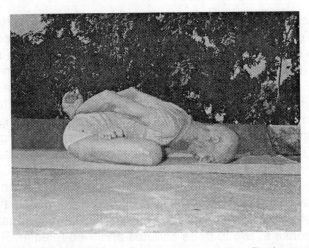

right thigh. In other words, assume the Padmasana posture. Keeping the head and spine erect, throw the hands to the back. With the left hand catch hold of the

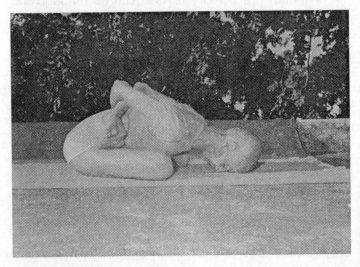

right wrist, behind the trunk. Exhale and slowly bend forward until the forehead touches the floor. Retain in this posture without inhalation, (or with normal breathing, whichever you feel comfortable) for ten seconds in the beginning. Concentrate on the forehead, abdomen and back muscles. Then, slowly return to the upright sitting position and release the hands. Gradually increase the duration from five to six minutes with normal breathing.

Variation: Instead of catching hold of the wrist, you may catch hold of the toes, the right toes by the right hand and the left toes by the left hand, as in the picture.

BENEFITS

This removes abdominal disorders and tones up the abdominal organs of secretion. This also intensifies the peristaltic activity, removes constipation and increases the digestive power. This Asana also helps to awaken the Kundalini Sakti.

18. MAYURASANA

(Peacock posture)

TECHNIQUE

Kneel on the floor with the knees slightly apart and the toes resting on the ground. Bend the body forward, join the arms together and rest the palms on the floor, with the two little fingers touching each other, and all the fingers pointing to the feet. Keep the arms firm, bent at the elbows. Let the forearms be kept close together.

Slowly bend forward and rest the abdomen on the elbows, and the chest on the upper part of the arms. Stretch the legs back one by one, and keep them to-

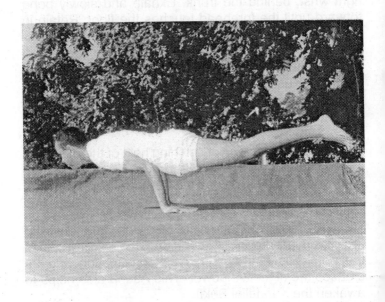

gether, stiff. Exhale and stretch your body, raising and keeping the legs straight. Secure balance and further stretch out the body parallel to the ground, and remain in the pose as long as you can comfortably. Retain the posture for a few seconds to start with. Gradually increase the duration to two or three minutes with normal breathing. To release from the pose, first lower the head and then the legs. Then place the knees by the side of the hands and thereafter release the position of the hands. Lie flat on the floor and relax in Savasana.

You would notice that your balance and the duration of stay in the Asana, increase as your wrists gradually gain strength.

Note: Beginners may find it difficult to maintain the balance when they raise the feet off the ground. Sometimes, they may have a fall forwards and may cause hurt to their nose. To avoid this, a cushion may be kept in front. When there is any difficulty to keep the balance, try to slip on the sides. In the final position, the head, trunk, legs and feet will be in one straight line, parallel to the ground.

BENEFITS

Besides strengthening the forearms, elbows and wrists, this Asana removes various abdominal diseases. It increases digestive power and tones up the stomach, kidneys and spleen. It is specially beneficial to those suffering from diabetes. Proper circulation of fresh blood is effected into the internal organs of the abdominal region.

19. SITTING POSTURES

(1) PADMASANA

(Lotus posture)

TECHNIQUE

Sit over a folded blanket placed on even floor, with stretched legs. Always keep the spine and neck erect without bend. This is an instruction common to all the sitting postures. Bend the right leg at the knee and place the right foot on the left thigh. Then, bend the left leg at the knee and place the left foot on the right thigh. Place the two hands with the palms facing up on the respective knee joints. Let the bent index fingers touch the middle portion of the thumbs and keep the other fingers stretched out. In the alternative, you can make the

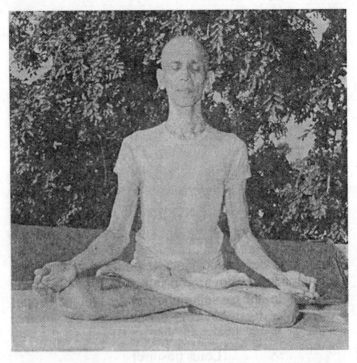

finger lock, and keep the locked hands over the left ankle. This may be convenient for some persons.

In the beginning, sit for ten minutes and gradually increase the duration according to your convenience.

(2) SIDDHASANA
(Adept's posture)

TECHNIQUE

Place one heel at the anus, the terminal opening of the alimentary canal or digestive tube. Keep the other

SITTING POSTURES

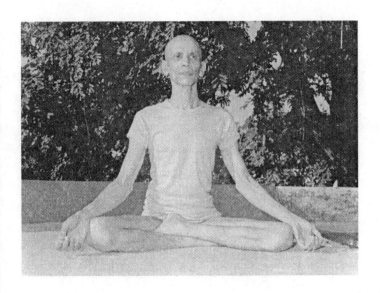

heel at the root of the generative organ. The feet and the legs should be so nicely arranged that the ankle-joints should touch each other. Hands can be placed as in Padmasana.

(3) SVASTIKASANA

(Crossed leg posture)

TECHNIQUE

Fold the left leg and place the feet near the right thigh muscles. Similarly, bend the right leg and push it

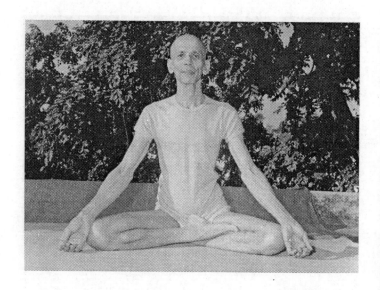

in the space between the left thigh and calf muscles. Now you find the two feet between the thighs and calves of the legs. Place the hands as in Padmasana.

(4) VAJRASANA
(Adamantine posture)

TECHNIQUE

Kneel on the floor, slowly rest the buttocks in between the heels. The calf muscles must touch the

SITTING POSTURES

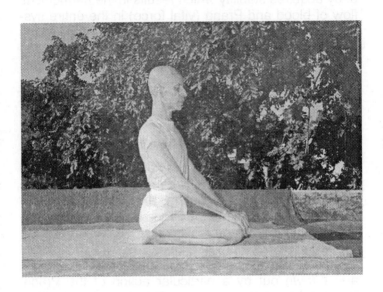

thighs. The parts from the toes to the knees should rest on the ground. The entire weight of the body should rest on the knees and ankles. In the beginning of the practice, you may feel a slight pain in the knee and ankle joints, but it will pass away by gradual practice. Place the left and right hand palms on the respective knees. Keep the spine and neck erect. This may be a comfortable sitting posture for many persons.

BENEFITS

By sitting in any one of the above postures, the body acquires stability which results in the harmonious flow of blood and Prana (vital force) in the entire system, which is prerequisite for meditation. These sitting postures strengthen the waist, tone up the nervous system and balance the vital forces. If one sits in this Vajrasana for about half an hour immediately after food, the food will be digested well. The nerves, muscles of the legs and thighs are strengthened.

20. PRANAYAMA

Regulation of Prana (vital force) is called Pranayama. The Prana is not merely the breath. The breathing process, (inhalation, exhalation and retention) does not constitute the Prana by itself, but is an indication that the Prana is working. We cannot see the Prana as it is not a physical object. But we can infer its existence from the process of respiration. Air is taken in and thrown out by a particular action of the Prana. Some hold that there are many Pranas and others think it is one. The Prana is really a single energy, but appears to be many when viewed from the standpoints of its different functions. Pranayama is a method of harmonising not only the breath, but also the senses and the mind. Through the practice of Pranayama, the body becomes strong and healthy. Too much of fat is reduced. There will be lusture in the face of the practitioner who will be free from diseases like cold, cough etc.

By the practice of Pranayama, the apices of the lungs will get proper supply of oxygen. There will be an improvement in the quality and quantity of the blood in the system. All the tissues and cells will be nourished with plenty of pure blood and lymph. The process of metabolism will be carried out in an efficient manner.

Important Note: (i) Pranayama exercises should be preceded by relaxation in Savasana, so that the body and mind may be calm and undisturbed before starting Pranayama.

(ii) All the Pranayama exercises should be practised in any one of the sitting postures with head, neck and spine erect.

(1) DEEP BREATHING EXERCISE

TECHNIQUE

After relaxing in Savasana, sit in any one of the sitting postures according to your convenience. Inhale and exhale through both the nostrils, without producing any sound. During inhalation, expand the chest and lungs and feel that fresh oxygen is entering the system, and during exhalation, contract the lungs as much as possible and also feel that all the impurities are going out.

If you feel that the nostrils are blocked due to cold, gently press the right nostril with the right thumb and breathe in; and breathe out through the left nostril, without producing any sound. Then close the left nostril with the help of the little and ring fingers of the right hand, slowly inhale and exhale through the right nostril, without producing any sound. Do this process six times. Gradually increase it to twelve times. This is one round. You can increase the number of rounds according to your strength and capacity.

BENEFITS

This clears the bronchial and nasal passages, frees one from cold, headache, etc., and increases the breathing capacity of the lungs.

(2) KAPALABHATI

(Skull cleaning exercise)

'Kapala' means skull and 'Bhati' means shine. This exercise cleanses the skull. Thus it becomes a purificatory exercise. The regular practice bestows a shining (skull) face to the practitioner. This prepares the student for the practice of Bhastrika Pranayama (see item 3 below).

TECHNIQUE

Sit in any one of the sitting postures and keep the spine and neck erect. Exhale quickly through the nostrils with a slight movement of the lower abdomen. Concentrate on the tip of the nose. You should not contract the face muscles. Short inhalation should follow each exhalation. To start with, you can have a speed of one expulsion per second and you can practise one or two rounds, each round consisting of eight or ten expulsions. Take rest with normal breaths after each round. When one is sufficiently advanced in the practice one can increase at the rate of ten expulsions for each round, per week, till one gets 120 expulsions in each round. Two or three rounds may be done in the morning and evening.

BENEFITS

This exercise cleanses the skull, the respiratory system and the nasal passages. It destroys diseases of the phlegm. It removes the spasm in the bronchial tubes. Consequently, Asthma is relieved and cured also. The impurities of the blood are thrown out. Heart functions properly. The circulatory, respiratory and digestive systems are toned up to a considerable degree.

(3) BHASTRIKA

(Rapid movement like that of the bellows)

Bhastrika means bellows. Rapid succession of forcible exhalations is a characteristic feature of the Pranayama.

TECHNIQUE

Sit in any of the postures. Rapid and deep expulsion and intake of breath through the nostrils should follow one another in quick succession. With each expulsion and inhalation of breath, contraction and expansion of abdomen should be there. Start with six, eight or ten expulsions of breath for one round, according to your capacity. The final expulsion in each round should follow with deep inhalation and retention of breath as long as you feel comfortable. Rest a while after one round of Bhastrika. Care should be taken that unnecessary pressure is not given on the lungs. Beginners may start with two or three rounds, each round consisting of six to ten expulsions, one expulsion per second. Gradually increase the number of the exhalation and inhalation to 20-30 per round, keeping the number of rounds to 2 or 3.

BENEFITS

Bhastrika relieves inflammation of the throat, increases the gastric fire, destroys accumulation of phlegm, removes the diseases of the nose and chest and eradicates asthma, constipation, excess of wind and bile. It gives warmth to the body. The practitioner will keep good health.

(4) SITALI
(Cooling Pranayama)

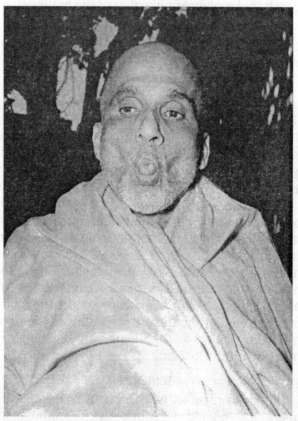

TECHNIQUE

Sit in any one of the postures. Open the mouth and form the lips into 'O' shape. Protrude the tongue like a tube. Draw in the air through the tongue tube. Fill the lungs with fresh and cool air as much as possible. After inhalation, withdraw the tongue and close the mouth. Lower your head and touch the collar bone with the chin during retention of breath. (For the Posture see page no. 84). Exhale slowly through both the nostrils after bringing your head erect. Practise this daily ten to fifteen times.

BENEFITS

This Pranayama cools the system, soothes the eyes and ears and purifies the blood. It quenches thirst and appeases hunger. It cures chronic dyspepsia (indigestion), inflammation of the spleen, various chronic skin diseases, low fever, biliousness and phlegm disorders.

(5) SITKARI

[Sound (seet) producing Pranayama]

TECHNIQUE

Open the mouth, fold the tongue upwards inside the mouth so that the tip of the tongue might touch the upper palate, and draw the air through the mouth with a hissing sound (seet). After inhalation, bring the tongue to its original position. Retain the breath as long as you feel comfortable, and then exhale slowly through the nostrils. Repeat it six times, and gradually increase the number.

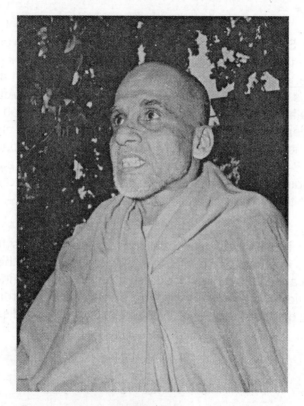

BENEFITS

Same as in Sitali Pranayama.

(6) UJJAYI
(Loud sound producing Pranayama)

TECHNIQUE

Sit in a comfortable posture. Close the mouth and eyes and concentrate on the sound produced during in-

PRANAYAMA

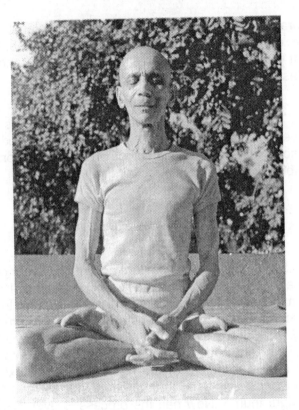

halation due to the partial closure of the glottis. Inhale through both the nostrils in a smooth, uniform manner. The sound produced during inhalation should be continuous and of uniform pitch. Expand the chest when you inhale. The passage of the incoming air is felt on the roof of the palate and makes a sibilant sound. Care should be taken not to bloat the abdomen in the process of inhalation. Then, exhale slowly, deeply and rhythmically through both the nostrils. After some days of practice, you can also exhale through the left nostril after closing the right nostril with the right thumb. Repeat the process five to ten times to start with, and increase the number according to your capacity.

BENEFITS

This Pranayama aerates the lungs, soothes the nerves and tones up the entire system. It is good for persons suffering from high blood pressure or coronary troubles, when done in a reclining position.

(7) SUKHA PURVAKA PRANAYAMA

(Easy comfortable breathing)

TECHNIQUE

Sit in a comfortable posture according to your convenience. Keep the spine, neck and head erect. Keep the middle and index fingers bent and the other three stretched. Close the right nostril with the right thumb. Very, very slowly inhale through the left nostril without producing any sound. Then close the left nostril with the little and ring fingers of the right hand. Then exhale very, very slowly through the right nostril, by releasing the right thumb. Now half the process is over. Slowly and harmoniously draw in air through the right nostril and exhale slowly through the left nostril. This completes one round. The ratio for inhalation and exhalation should be 1:2. During the first fifteen days inhale for 5 seconds and exhale for 10 seconds. In the second fortnight increase the duration of time to ten seconds for inhalation and twenty seconds for exhalation. During inhalation and exhalation, expand and contract (respectively) the lungs, as much as possible.

PRANAYAMA

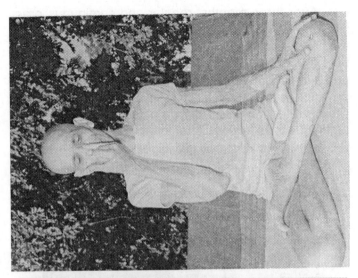

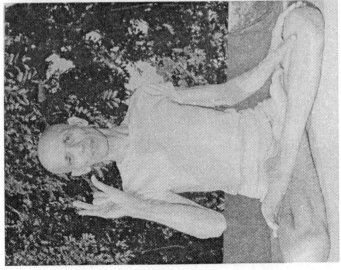

After three months' regular and continuous practice, you can introduce retention of breath. The ratio in the time for inhalation, retention and exhalation should be 1:2:2, i.e., if you inhale for 5 seconds, the retention and exhalation should be for 10 seconds each. As you advance in the practice, you may adopt the ratio 1:4:2. During retention, you may do Jalandhara Bandha. Its technique is as follows. After inhalation, slowly bend the

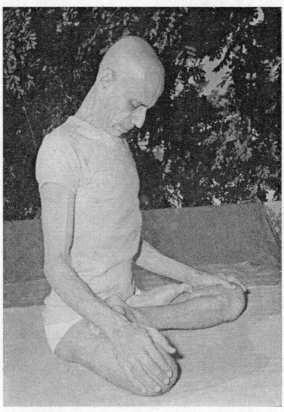

neck and rest the chin on the collar bone while retaining the breath. This Bandha prevents the pressure of air moving upwards, towards the head. (For the Posture see previous page)

Before exhalation, slowly lift the head, keep it erect, and then exhale. This is release of Jalandhara Bandha.

Warning: If you feel headache, heaviness of the head, giddiness, uneasiness, etc., it means, you are exerting and giving much pressure on the lungs. You should therefore reduce the duration of time of retention. The first symptom of correct practice of Pranayama is, the feeling of freshness, energy and lightness of the body and mind. If you feel any negative result, avoid the practice of retention of breath immediately and consult an expert.

BENEFITS

This Pranayama removes all diseases, purifies the Nadis, steadies the mind in concentration, increases the digestive fire and appetite, helps to maintain Brahmacharya.

(21) DHYANA

(Meditation)

Meditation is the seventh limb according to the Yoga Sutras of sage Patanjali, the eighth being Samadhi. There are many methods of practice of concentration which leads to meditation. The purpose of meditation is to understand the real nature of the object of meditation. The mind is the instrument with which we meditate. A certain amount of the study of the nature of activities of the mind is necessary before one takes up

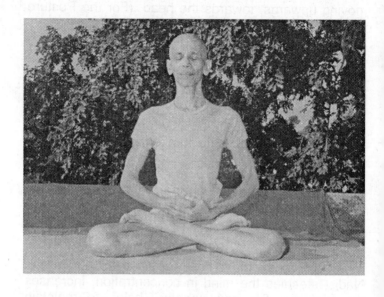

to meditation. The existence of the mind can be found only during its activities. The thief can be found out only during the act of thieving, for at all other times he may look like an ordinary person. When the thief comes to know that the police are after him, he restricts his movements. Similarly, if you begin to study the mind, the mental processes or the activities of the mind will be reduced. There are mainly two stages of meditation. They are: (1) Constantly thinking on one object or thought, to

DHYANA

the exclusion of all other objects and thoughts; and (2) keeping the mind free of all thoughts.

In the first stage one must concentrate one's mind on an object, or engage oneself in the repetition of the Mantra into which he is initiated by his preceptor. If one starts repeating the Mantra with concentration on the Mantra, then alone one will come to know the innumerable other thoughts which lie submerged in one's subconscious and unconscious levels of the mind and which rise to the conscious level and cause disturbance to concentration on the Mantra. When the concentration on one Mantra together with Bhava (feeling of its meaning), is increased through a long and continued practice, the mind reaches the state of meditation.

In the second stage, one should sit in a comfortable posture, close the eyes and relax all the limbs of the body from toes to the crown of the head. The ears being open, external sounds naturally will impinge on them. One should be a witness to these external sounds and also be a witness to the inner thoughts that may arise one after another in endless succession. One should not go after those inner thoughts, nor should one pay any serious attention to the external sounds. By complete relaxation in the sitting posture and by remaining as a witness of the internal and external activities of the mind, the mind will become non-objectified, after continued, unbroken practice for a long period. In the early stages care should be taken that one does not go to sleep. Sincerity, earnestness and purity of thought, word and deed, are the important factors for success in the practice of meditation.

22. CONCLUSION

The purpose of Yoga is to create harmony in the physical, vital, mental, psychological and spiritual aspects of the human being. In the foregoing pages of this book, I have described the technique of relaxation in different postures viz., standing, lying and sitting postures which brings in this harmony. Yoga is not mere practice for an hour or two in a day but it is the most scientific way of living, all the twenty-four hours of the day. During the whole day you may be only in one of these three postures and hence a skilful adjustment in them will effect the required harmony. *"Yogasthah kuru karmani—* Be established in Yoga and do all your duties." *"Yogah karmasu kausalam—*Yoga is skill in action." Skill here means to be in tune with the nature of the Supreme Reality. Be a Yogin always, is the loving instruction of Lord Krishna. Convert life into Yoga, so that you may ensure success in all the fields of activity. By regular practice, by using your presence of mind, skill and wisdom, you can become Yogins and enjoy happiness and peace, whatever be the circumstances and conditions in which you are placed.

May the Grace of Gurudev Sri Swami Sivanandaji Maharaj and the Almighty be ever upon you all!

For more details on various Yoga Asanas, Pranayamas and Bandha Traya, and Meditation, kindly refer to the books: 'Yoga Asanas', 'The Science of Pranayama', and 'Concentration and Meditation' by Sri Swami Sivananda.

APPENDIX

APPENDIX

Appendix

BRIEF LIFE-SKETCH OF
SRI SWAMI CHIDANANDA

Sridhar Rao, as Swami Chidananda was known before taking Sannyasa, was born to Srinivasa Rao and Sarojini, on the 24th September 1916, the second of five children and the eldest son. Sri Srinivasa Rao was a prosperous Zamindar owning several villages, extensive lands and palatial buildings in South India. Sarojini was an ideal Indian mother, noted for her saintliness.

At the age of eight, Sridhar Rao's life was influenced by one Sri Anantayya, a friend of his grandfather, who used to relate to him stories from the epics, the Ramayana and the Mahabharata. Doing Tapas, becoming a Rishi, and having a vision of the Lord became ideals which he cherished.

His uncle, Krishna Rao, shielded him against the evil influences of the materialistic world around him, and sowed in him the seeds of the Nivritti life which he joyously nurtured until, as latter events proved, it blossomed into sainthood.

His elementary education began at Mangalore. In 1932 he joined the Muthiah Chetty School in Madras (now Chennai) where he distinguished himself as a brilliant student. His cheerful personality, exemplary conduct and extraordinary traits earned for him a distinct place in the hearts of all teachers and students with whom he came into contact.

In 1936, he was admitted to Loyola College, whose portals admit only the most brilliant of students. In 1938, he emerged with the degree of Bachelor of Arts. This period of studentship at a predominantly Christian College was significant. The glorious ideal of Lord Jesus, the Apostles and the other Christian saints had found in his heart a synthesis of all that is best and noble in the Hindu culture. To him, study of the Bible was no more routine; it was the living word of God, just as living and real as the words of the Vedas, the Upanishads and the Bhagavadgita. His innate breadth of vision enabled him to see Jesus in Krishna, not Jesus instead of Krishna. He was as much an adorer of Jesus Christ as he was of Lord Vishnu.

The family was noted for its high code of conduct and this was infused into his life. Charity and service were the glorious ingrained virtues of the members of the family. These virtues found an embodiment in Sridhar Rao. He discovered ways and means of manifesting them. None who sought his help was sent away without it. He gave freely to the needy.

Service to lepers became his ideal. He would build them huts on the vast lawn of his home and look after them as though they were deities. Later, after he joined the Ashram, this early trait found in him complete and free expression where even the best among men would seldom venture into this great realm of divine love, based upon the supreme wisdom that all are one in God. Patients from the neighbourhood, suffering from the worst kinds of diseases came to him. To Sridhar Rao the patient was none other than Lord Narayana Himself. He served him with tender love and compassion. The very movement of his hands portrayed him as worshipping the living Lord Narayana. Nothing would keep him from bringing comfort to the suffering inmates of the Ashram, no matter what the urgency of other engagements at the time.

Service, especially of the sick, often brought out the fact that he had no idea of his own separate existence as an individual. It seemed as if his body clung loosely to his soul.

Nor was all this service confined to human beings. Birds and animals claimed his attention as much as, if not more than, human beings. He understood their language of suffering. His service of a sick dog evoked the admiration of Gurudev. He would raise his finger in grim admonition when he saw anyone practising cruelty to dumb animals in his presence.

His deep and abiding interest in the welfare of lepers had earned for him the confidence and admiration of the Government authorities when he was elected to the Leper Welfare Association, constituted by the state—at first as Vice-Chairman and later as Chairman of the Muni-ki-reti Notified Area Committee.

Quite early in life, although born in a wealthy family, he shunned the pleasures of the world to devote himself to seclusion and contemplation. In the matter of study it was the spiritual books which had the most appeal to him, more than college books. Even while he was at the college, textbooks had to take second place to spiritual books. The works of Sri Ramakrishna, Swami Vivekananada and Sri Gurudev took precedence over all others. He shared his knowledge with others, so much so that he virtually became the Guru of the household and the neighbourhood, to whom he would talk of honesty, love, purity, service and devotion to God. He would exhort them to perform Japa of Rama-Nama. While still in his twenties he began initiating youngsters into this great Rama Taraka Mantra. He was an ardent admirer of Sri Ramakrishna Math at Madras and regularly participated in the Satsangas there. The call of Swami Vivekananda to renounce resounded within his pure heart. He ever thirsted for the Darshan of saints and Sadhus visiting the metropolis.

In June 1936, he disappeared from home. After a vigorous search by his parents, he was found in the secluded Ashram of a holy sage some miles from the sacred mountain shrine of Tirupati. He returned home after some persuasion. This temporary separation was but a preparation for the final parting from the world of attachments to family and friends. While at home his heart dwelt in silent forest of spiritual thoughts, beating in tune with the eternal Pranava-Nada of the Jnana Ganga within himself. The seven years at home following his return from Tirupati were marked by seclusion, service, intense study of spiritual literature, self-restraint, control of the senses, simplicity in food and dress, abandonment of all comforts and practice of austerities which augmented his inner spiritual power.

The final decision came in 1943. He was already in correspondence with Sri Swami Sivanandaji Maharaj of Rishikesh. He obtained Swamiji's permission to join the Ashram.

On arrival at the Ashram, he naturally took charge of the dispensary. He became the man with the healing hand. The growing reputation of his divine healing hand attracted a rush of patients to the Sivananda Charitable Dispensary.

Very soon after joining the Ashram, he gave ample evidence of the brilliance of his intellect. He delivered lectures, wrote articles for magazines and gave spiritual instructions to the visitors. When the Yoga-Vedanta Forest University (now known as the Yoga-Vedanta Forest Academy) was established in 1948, Sri Gurudev paid him a fitting tribute by appointing him Vice-Chancellor and Professor of Raja Yoga. During the first year he inspired the students with his brilliant exposition of Maharshi Patanjali's Yoga-Sutras.

It was also in the first year of his stay at the Ashram that he wrote his *magnum opus*, 'Light Fountain', an immortal biography of Sri Gurudev. Sri Gurudev himself once remarked: "Sivananda will pass away, but 'Light Fountain' will live."

In spite of his multifarious activities and intense Sadhana he founded, under the guidance of Gurudev, the Yoga Museum in 1947, in which the entire philosophy of Vedanta and all the processes of Yoga Sadhana are depicted in the form of pictures and illustrations.

Towards the end of 1948, Gurudev nominated him as General Secretary of the Divine Life Society. The great responsibility of the organisation fell on his shoulders. From that moment he spiritualised all its activities by his presence, counsel and wise leadership. He exhorted all to raise their consciousness to the level of the Divine.

On Guru Purnima day, the 10th of July, 1949, he was initiated into the holy order of Sanyasa by Sri

Swami Sivanandaji Maharaj. He now became known as Swami Chidananda, a name which connotes, "one who is in the highest consciousness and bliss".

In November, 1959, Swami Chidanandaji embarked on an extensive tour of America, being sent by Gurudev as his personal representative to broadcast the message of Divine Life. He returned in March, 1962.

In August 1963, after the Mahasamadhi of the Master, he was elected as the President of The Divine Life Society. After election, he strove to hold aloft the banner of renunciation, dedicated service, love and spiritual idealism, not only within the set-up of the widespread organisation of the Society, but in the hearts of countless seekers throughout the world, who were all too eager to seek his advice, help and guidance.

Sri Swami Chidanandaji has toured the length and breadth of India, Malaysia and South Africa to serve the devotees of the Society.

Again in 1968, Sri Swami Chidanandaji undertook the Global Tour at the kind request of numerous disciples and devotees of holy Master Sri Swami Sivanandaji Maharaj and visited all countries of the world. Wherever he went devotees received him cordially and listened to him with rapt attention.

Sri Swami Chidanandaji, right from the beginning was working and serving the Divine Cause of Sri Gurudev's Mission tirelessly and spreading his Divine Life Message far and wide not only in Bharatavarsha but also in countries outside.

APPENDIX

On the 24th of September, 1991 the Headquarters of The Divine Life Society Shivanandanagar (Rishikesh) as well as all Branches of the Society celebrated his 75th Birthday Anniversary *(Amritamahotsava).*

Swamiji Maharaj attained Mahasamadhi on 28th August, 2008.

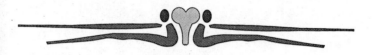